CONTENTS

Introduction
What is Inflammation?

Inflammation is a natural process that deals with stress or damage to the body. It is an essential part of the healing process that protects and repairs wounds following by harm, trauma, toxins or an attack of infection, bacteria or viruses. Inflammation happens by increasing the flow of white cells to the damaged cells that allows helpful antibodies to aid in healing by washing away the damage. A common example of inflammation around an injury or wound is

- Heat
- Pain
- Swelling
- Redness

You can observe inflammation on your injured skin section when it heats up slightly or gets red. And, thus, the skin becomes inflamed.

To put it simply, inflammation is a series of signals and defense mechanisms for the area of damage by anti-inflammatory cells. Then these cells trigger other cell and protective mechanisms and so on, and you know it, you are swelling, pain, and sometimes puss, which are just over-amplified reactions to the threat or harm.

In other words, cellular destruction is the first phase of inflammation, and then the second phase begins, which is cellular rejuvenation. These two phases need to be balanced, but the balance never happens due to our poor diet lifestyle. The trans-fats, grains, and sugar trigger inflammatory immune response, and this means every time we eat these foods, we are inflaming our bodies over and over again. As a result, the immune system gets out of control and causes excess inflammation for a longer time, or when it triggers inflammation when it is not necessary.

Though there are many things to do to lower inflammation; however, for long-term health, eating healthy is crucial. And, that's the goal of an anti-inflammatory diet.

What is Anti-Inflammation Diet?

An anti-inflammation Diet or AI diet focuses on fighting with chronic inflammation by eating certain healthy foods and avoiding those foods that can cause it. As mentioned before that inflammation is a natural process, but it can occur by mistakes and causes adverse health effects, which leads to inflammatory diseases like

- heart disease
- arthritis
- diabetes
- fatty liver disease
- Alzheimer's disease
- Parkinson diseases
- kidney failure
- loss of function of muscles
- swelling
- breast cancer

In fact, misplaced inflammation can affect any organ. When this happens, the immune system becomes overactive by enhancing blood flow and sending surplus cells unnecessary that cause swelling, pain, and heat where there has been no trauma and infection. It's is also known as autoimmunity, and that's when the body attached itself without external injury or assault.

The overall effect of inflammation and its seriousness depends on how long it lasts. Short term inflammation is generally resolved entirely and leave no problems. But, long term or chronic inflammation may last several months to years and may cause severe and lasting damage to the organs or infection.

How Do You Get Inflammation?

Chronic inflammation can happen to anyone, but people who are overweight, obese, or under stress have more risks of inflammation. People who have an inactive lifestyle or those who do a lot of sitting can promote inflammation.

What's more, eating foods that have high sugar content, refined grains, saturated fats, gluten, dairy, processed meats, packaged foods, and drinking alcohol contributes to inflammation. The use of vegetable oil and excessive intake of alcohol are another possible culprit.

Toxins in environments or air pollution also trigger the immune system this way that causes excess inflammation.

Signs of Chronic Inflammation

How does one know that s/he have inflammation. The following are some signs, and if you have one of these symptoms, you might be affected by inflammation.

- Frequent headaches
- Brain fog
- Fatigue
- Bloating
- Weight gain
- Digestive problems
- Allergies
- Joint pains
- Rashes
- Gum diseases
- Mood swings

The Role of Diet

So if you want to reduce inflammation, you need to eat well rather than doing worse with a poor diet. For this, you need to plan your diet with whole, nutritionally dense and anti-inflammatory friendly foods and avoid inflammatory foods. The anti-inflammatory foods are packed with antioxidants, which reduces levels of free radicals that are created and part of metabolism and can leads to inflammation when they are not held in check.

Each meal of anti-inflammatory diet contains a healthy balance of fat, carbs, and protein, and it also makes sure that the body meets its regular requirement of fiber, water, minerals, and vitamins as well.

One diet that is considered anti-inflammatory is the traditional Mediterranean diet. The foods comprise of vegetables, fruits, legumes, whole-grains, fatty fish, and olive oil have proved to lower inflammatory markers such as interleukin-6 (IL-6) and C-reactive protein (CRP) in the blood compared to those who don't. Also, low-carb diets significantly reduce inflammation by shedding weight for people who have are obese. Vegetarian and vegan diets are also linked to reducing inflammation.

The goals of the anti-inflammatory diet are simple that is cutting back on foods that can trigger inflammation and eat more foods that heal the injuries and damage in the body. While there are some variations in what to avoid and eat, most of the anti-inflammatory diet plans emphasize on eating whole foods comprises of non-starchy veggies, fruits, berries, mono-saturated fats like avocado and olive oil, lots of fatty fish and avoiding refined grains, highly processed and deep-fried foods, and added sugar.

Foods to Fight Inflammation

The focus of the AI diet is to maintain the balance of macronutrients from fats, proteins, and carbohydrates. The calories of anti-inflammatory food should contain 30 percent fats, 20 – 30 percent protein, and 40 – 50 percent carbohydrates.

What Can I Eat?

Healthy Carbs:
- Grains: Eat whole grains such as brown rice, quinoa, whole-grain pasta, and loaves of bread. Use gluten-free flours for baking like almond flour, coconut flour, brown rice flour, buckwheat flour, etc.
- Vegetables: Consume fresh and organic vegetables that are high in fiber such as dark leafy greens, like kale, spinach, lettuce, tomatoes, mushrooms, bell peppers, onion, carrots, ginger, olives, avocado, sweet potatoes, winter squash and cauliflower, cabbage, Brussel sprouts, Bok Choi, arugula, eggplant, okra, etc.
- Fruits: Opt for high-fat and antioxidant-rich fruits like apple, grapes, oranges, apricots, banana, cherry, blueberries, strawberries, and cherries.

Healthy Fats:
- Oils: Opt for healthy unsaturated fats and plant-based oil for cooking such as olive oil, avocado oil, coconut oil, grapeseed oil, canola oil, sunflower oil, safflower oil, etc. Use plant-based butter like coconut butter and almond butter.
- Nuts and seeds: Incorporates nuts into the meals like almonds, cashews, Brazil nuts, Macadamia nuts, and walnuts as they contain healthy fats. Use seeds such as sesame seeds, sunflower seeds, pumpkin seeds, flaxseeds, hemp seeds, chia seeds, etc.
- Fish: Eat omega-3 fatty acids riched foods like wild-caught fatty fishes such as tuna, anchovies, salmon, mackerel, sardines, black cod, oysters, shrimps, etc.
- Cheese: Consume low-fat cheeses like parmesan cheese, cottage cheese, mozzarella cheese, cheddar cheese, etc.

Healthy Proteins:
- Beans: Get plant-based proteins from beans such as kidney beans, chickpeas, lentils, and pulses.
- Soy products: Eat tofu, tempeh, and other vegan meat alternates to meet your protein requirements than animal products.
- Poultry: Get protein from pasture-raised poultry like chicken, turkey, lamb, hens, etc.
- Dairy: Pastured eggs, unsweetened, or plain Greek yogurt are great options for protein.

Healthy Drinks:
- Water: Drink water as much as you want. You can also drink lemon water or lemonade as well.
- Tea: Drink unsweetened and low-fat tea and coffee, green tea, turmeric tea, and herbal tea.
- Alcohol: Drink red wine in moderation, about 10 ounces per day for men, and 5 ounces per day for women.

Spices and Sweeteners:

- Chocolate: Eat dark chocolate in moderate to satisfy your sweet tooth.
- Plant-based sweeteners: Other options to add sweetness in foods are coconut sugar, stevia, erythritol, etc.
- Spices: Incorporate spices in your foods that are known for anti-inflammatory properties like turmeric, ginger, cinnamon, rosemary, thyme, sage, cloves, curry powder, cumin seeds, cayenne pepper, cloves, coriander,

What's Off the Menu?

Carbs:
- White starches
- Refined grains
- White bread
- White pasta
- Package snacks
- Baked goods such as cookies, pastries, and cake
- Ready-made meals, curries, and sauces
- Deep-fried foods like French fries

Fats:
- Hydrogenated and processed seed oils like corn oil, soybean oil, etc.
- Processed foods like chips, crackers, pretzels, etc.
- Full-fat butter
- Full-fat cream
- Milk with added sugar
- High-fat cheese
- High-fat yogurt
- Palm oil
- Margarine
- Shortening
- Lard

Proteins:
- Fatty cuts of meats like red meat
- Processed meats such as sausages, hot dogs, etc.

Drinks:
- Sodas
- Beverages with added sugar
- Sweetened fruit juiced
- Sweetened drinks
- Excessive alcohol

Sweetness
- Table sugar
- Candies
- Ice cream

Rules of Anti-Inflammatory Diet

Following are some principles you should follow on the anti-inflammatory diet

- **Eat a minimum of 25g fiber every day.**

Fiber riched foods supply natural anti-inflammatory nutrients, which helps in lowering inflammation. Therefore, focus on consuming more vegetables, fruits, and other whole foods that are abundant in fiber. The best sources of fiber include vegetables like onion, eggplant, okra, fruits like banana, and blueberries.

- **Eat at least nine servings of veggies and fruits every day.**

Here one serving means 1 cup of raw leafy greens or ½ cup of cooked vegetable or fruits. You can add extra flavor to your cooked vegetables and fruits by incorporating anti-inflammatory herbs and spices like ginger and turmeric to increase their antioxidant levels.

- **Eat four servings of crucifers and allium every week.**

Alliums refer to vegetables that include leeks, scallion, onion, and garlic, while crucifers include vegetables like mustard greens, cabbage, broccoli, cauliflower, and Brussel sprouts. These groups of vegetables have powerful anti-oxidant properties, and therefore, it is recommended to consume them about four servings weekly. It significantly helps in lowering the risks of cancer.

- **Limit daily intake of saturated fat to 10 percent of calories.**

Keeping the saturated fat lower in your foods will help in reducing the risk of heart diseases. In addition, limit the red meat to one time in a well and then omit it from your meals. And, when you have meat in a meal, marinate it with anti-inflammatory spices, herbs, and fruit juices to lower its toxic compounds that are formed during cooking.

- **Consume Omega-3 fatty acid foods more.**

It has proven that foods that are abundant in omega-3 fatty acids lower inflammation and reduce the risk of chronic diseases. Moreover, other options to eat omega-3 fatty acids like kidney, soy, navy beans, walnuts, and flax meal. And, consume lots of fatty fishes like anchovies, salmon, sardines, oysters, etc., at least thrice a week.

- **Use oils that are high in healthy fats.**

Your body needs fats, but for this, choose fats that are healthy and provide the body with benefits. For example, olive oil, avocado oil, sunflower oil, and other organic plant-based oils are the best options for anti-inflammatory benefits.

- **Eat healthy snacks twice a day.**

Snacking is a great way to fill your tummy with healthy and nutritious fruits, rather than going on a food strike to lose weight and maintain health. Go for fruits, baby carrots, celery sticks, unsweetened yogurt, almonds, walnuts, and pistachios.

- **Avoid refined sugars and processed foods.**

Foods that are high in sodium like snacks and high in sugar like corn syrup and artificial sweeteners contribute to inflammation, so avoid them wherever possible. Along with raising inflammation in the body, refined sugar also causes fatty liver disease, diabetes, increase the uric acid level and blood pressure, and more.

- **Cut out trans fats.**

Research has proved that foods that contain trans fats increase the levels of C-reactive protein, which is a biomarker for inflammation. Therefore, you need to put away products from your pantry that contain the words "partially hydrogenated oil" or "hydrogenated oil" in the food labels like margarine, crackers, shortening, cookies, etc.

Ginger Tea

"Begin your day with a nourishing and warming cup of ginger tea. You can enjoy this anti-inflammatory drink at any time of the day."

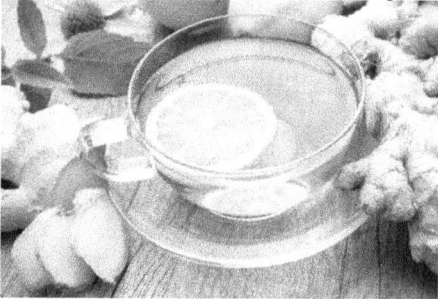

Prep Time: -5minutes -Calories: -7.5
Cook Time: -15minutes -Fat (g): -0 g
Total Time: -20minutes -Protein (g): -0.1 g
Servings: -1 -Carbs (g): -2.4 g

Ingredients:

Fresh ginger, peeled and sliced -1, about 2 inches
Water -2 cups
Lemon juice -2 tablespoons
Cinnamon -¼ teaspoon

Instructions:

1.   Place a saucepan over medium heat, pour in water, add ginger and then bring it to light-boil.
2.   Cover the pan, continue boiling the water for 15 minutes and then remove the saucepan from heat.
3.   Strain the mixture in a mug, remove the ginger pieces, add lemon juice into the tea and stir in cinnamon until combined.
4.   Serve straight away.

Herbal Chamomile Tea

"Ginger is an immunity-boosting ingredient, and its pair with lemon and rosemary makes an incredible health tonic. Drinking this tea will help you boost your immune system and lowers the inflammation."

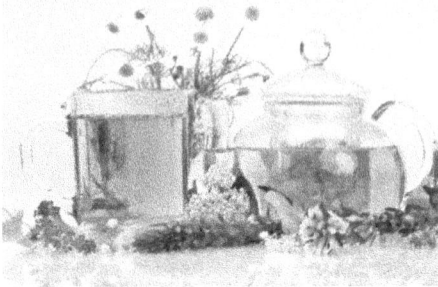

Prep Time: -25minutes -Calories: -6
Cook Time: -0minutes -Fat (g): -0 g
Total Time: -25minutes -Protein (g): -0 g
Servings: -4 -Carbs (g): -1 g

Ingredients:
Grated ginger, fresh -Two teaspoons
Slices of lemon -4
Chamomile tea -Six bags
Honey -Four teaspoons
Rosemary -Two sprigs
Boiling water -4 cups

Instructions:
1.   Pour boiling water in a large heatproof bowl, add ginger, lemon, and rosemary and stir in honey.
2.   Add tea bags and let them steep in the water for 20 minutes, stirring occasionally.
3.   Strain the liquid between four mugs, pressing the teabags to take out liquid as much as possible and then serve.

Matcha Green Tea Latte

"This creamy latte features the right balance between honey and bitterness of match. Have this healthy latte tea alternate to tea and coffee."

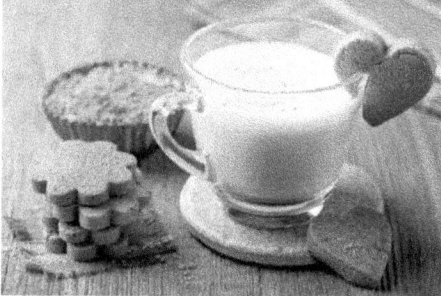

Prep Time: -5minutes -Calories: -124
Cook Time: -5minutes -Fat (g): -2 g
Total Time: -10minutes -Protein (g): -8 g
Servings: -1 -Carbs (g): -18 g

Ingredients:

Matcha tea powder -One teaspoon
Honey -One teaspoon
Almond milk, low-fat -1 cup
Boiling water -¼ cup

Instructions:

1. Pour boiling water in a blender, add matcha tea powder and then pulse until foamy.
2. Pour milk in a small saucepan, bring it to a light boil, and then whisking continuously until frothy.
3. Pour the heated milk in a mug, add tea mixture and stir well until combined.
4. Serve straight away.

Turmeric Latte

"Turmeric is known for its amazing benefits to the body, specifically reducing inflammation. And, this healthy turmeric latte recipe is a perfect way to take all the advantages of turmeric."

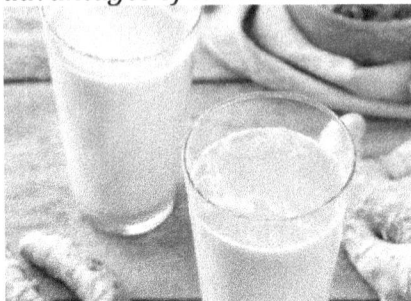

Prep Time: -10minutes -Calories: -70
Cook Time: -30minutes -Fat (g): -3 g
Total Time: -40minutes -Protein (g): -1 g
Servings: -1 -Carbs (g): -11 g

Ingredients:

Honey -Two teaspoons
Fresh ginger, grated -One teaspoon
Ground pepper -1/16 teaspoon
Ground cinnamon-1/8 teaspoon
Fresh turmeric, grated -One tablespoon
Almond milk, unsweetened -1 cup

Instructions:

1. Pour milk in a blender, then add remaining ingredients except for cinnamon and pulse until blended and very smooth.
2. Pour the mixture into a small saucepan, place the pan over medium-high heat and cook for 3 minutes or more until steaming hot.
3. Pour the mixture into a mug, garnish with cinnamon and serve.

Beet and Kale Smoothie

"This purple smoothie is abundant with lots of taste and anti-inflammatory nutrients like fiber, mineral, and vitamins. It will help your body a lot in healing and calming. It is so easy to make, and you can even take it with you. "

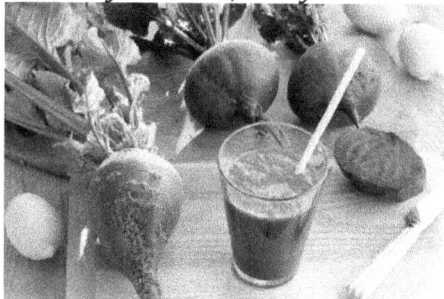

Prep Time: -5minutes -Calories: -264
Cook Time: -0minutes -Fat (g): -8 g
Total Time: -5minutes -Protein (g): -5 g
Servings: -2 -Carbs (g): -47 g
Ingredients:
Baby kale -2 cups
Small beet, peeled, chopped -1
Fresh ginger, grated -One tablespoon
Orange, peeled -1
Strawberry, frozen -2/3 cup
Blueberry, frozen -2/3 cup
Blackberry, frozen -2/3 cup
Pineapple, frozen -1 cup
Water -1 cup
Coconut oil -One tablespoon
Instructions:
1.   Place kale in a blender, add beet and orange, pour in water, and pulse until puree and smooth.
2.   Add remaining ingredients and then continue blending until smooth.
3.   Divide the smoothie between two glasses and serve.

Blueberry Hemp Seed Smoothie

"This recipe features another smoothie that has nourishing anti-inflammatory foods. Have it for breakfast or enjoy it as an energizing snack or even meal."

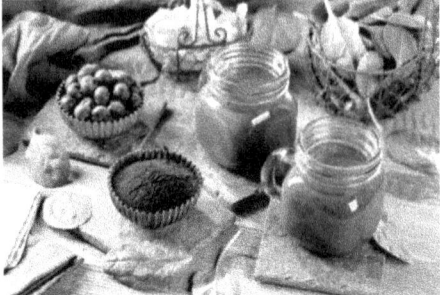

Prep Time: -5minutes -Calories: -112
Cook Time: -0minutes -Fat (g): -1.1 g
Total Time: -5minutes -Protein (g): -2.1 g
Servings: -1 -Carbs (g): -27 g
Ingredients:
Blueberries, frozen -1 ¼ cup
Kale -1/2 cup
Hemp seeds -Two tablespoons
Vanilla protein powder, plant-based -1 scoop
Basil powder -1/4 teaspoon
Spirulina-1 teaspoon
Almond milk, unsweetened -One ¼ cup
Instructions:
1. Place all the ingredients in a blender and pulse until puree and smooth.
2. Pour the smoothie in a glass and serve.

Greek Yogurt Smoothie

"Greek yogurt smoothie is perfect for reenergizing you after your workout. Moreover, it will also help in reducing and discomfort or swelling caused by exercise."

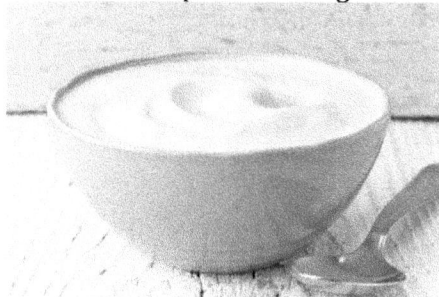

Prep Time: -5minutes -Calories: -171.3
Cook Time: -0minutes -Fat (g): -1.5 g
Total Time: -5minutes -Protein (g): -6.3 g
Servings: -1 -Carbs (g): -35.4 g
Ingredients:
Baby spinach -¼ cup
Ground cinnamon -1/8 teaspoon
Almond butter -One tablespoon
Greek yogurt -½ cup
Almond milk, unsweetened -1 cup
Ice cubes -4
Instructions:
1. Place all the ingredients in a blender and pulse until puree and smooth.
2. Pour the smoothie in a glass and serve.

Rhubarb, Apple and Ginger Muffin

"The combination of rhubarb, ginger, and apple are the star ingredients in this recipe, which take classical muffin to a new level of taste. Moreover, these foods are high in antioxidants, which make these muffin anti-inflammatory friendly foods."

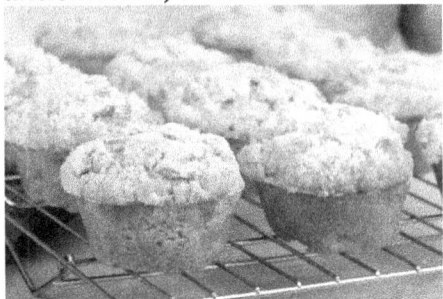

Prep Time: -15minutes -Calories: -221
Cook Time: -25minutes -Fat (g): -13 g
Total Time: -40minutes -Protein (g): -5 g
Servings: -8 -Carbs (g): -21 g

Ingredients:

Almond meal -1/2 cup
Ground linseed meal -One tablespoon
Coconut sugar -1/4 cup
Crystallized ginger, chopped -Two tablespoons
Buckwheat flour -1/2 cup
Brown rice flour -1/4 cup
Arrowroot -Two tablespoons
Baking powder -Two teaspoons
Ground ginger -1/2 teaspoon
Ground cinnamon -1/2 teaspoon
Sea salt -1/16 teaspoon
Small apple, peeled, cored, diced -1
Rhubarb, sliced -1 cup
Vanilla extract, unsweetened -One teaspoon
Olive oil -1/4 cup
Almond milk, unsweetened -1/3 cup and one tablespoon
Egg, pastured -1

Instructions:

1. Switch on the oven, set it to 350 degrees F, and let preheat.
2. Meanwhile, place the almond meal in a bowl, add linseed meal and stir in ginger and sugar until combined.
3. Add rice flour and buckwheat flour along with arrowroot, baking powder, and ginger, cinnamon, and salt; stir until well mixed and then fold in rhubarb and apple until just combined.
4. Crack the egg in another bowl, whisk in vanilla, oil, and milk until blended and then pour into the flour mixture and whisk well until incorporated and smooth batter comes together.
5. Take an eight cups muffin pan, line the cups with muffin tins, and evenly fill with prepared batter and bake the muffins in the oven for 20 to 25 minutes until the top of muffins is browned and inserted skewer into each muffin slide out clean.
6. When muffins have baked, let them cool in the pan for 5 minutes and then transfer them to a wire rack to cool completely.
7. Serve straight away.

Gingerbread Oatmeal

"Oatmeal is high in fiber, and this protects the body against colon cancer. Take advantage of these amazing properties and more with this gingerbread oatmeal bowl."

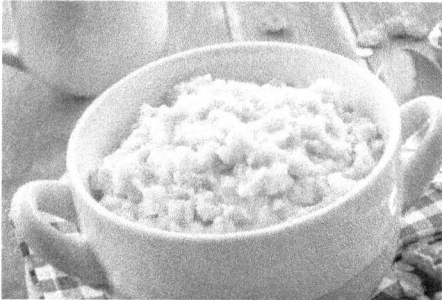

Prep Time: -5minutes -Calories: -158
Cook Time: -15minutes -Fat (g): -3.2 g
Total Time: -20minutes -Protein (g): -6 g
Servings: -4 -Carbs (g): -27 g

Ingredients:
Oats, steel-cut -1 cup
Ground ginger -1/4 teaspoon
Ground cinnamon -1 ½ tablespoon
Ground cardamom -1/4 teaspoon
Ground coriander -1/4 teaspoon
Ground cloves -1/4 teaspoon
Ground allspice -1/4 teaspoon
Ground nutmeg -1/8 teaspoon
Water -4 cups

Instructions:
1.   Take a medium saucepan, pour in water, place it over medium-high heat and then bring to boil.
2.   Then reduce heat to medium-low, add oats, add remaining ingredients, stir until mixed and cook for 5 to 10 minutes or until oats have softened and most of the liquid is absorbed.
3.   When oats have cooked, remove the pan from the heat, cover the pan and let it stand for 3 minutes.
4.   Evenly divide the oats into four bowls, drizzle with maple syrup, top with favorite fruit, and serve.

Cherry Coconut Porridge

"Decadent cherry and coconut porridge is a wonderful treat for your taste buds as a breakfast, snack or dessert. Make ahead and have it any time of the day."

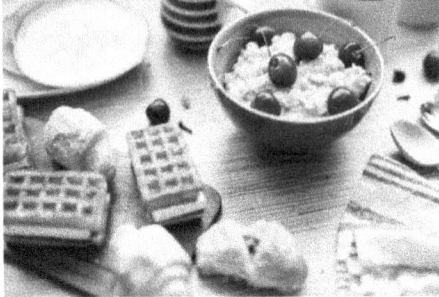

Prep Time: -5minutes -Calories: -402
Cook Time: -15minutes -Fat (g): -22 g
Total Time: -20minutes -Protein (g): -7.6 g
Servings: -1 -Carbs (g): -44 g

Ingredients:
Oats, steel-cut -1 ½ cup
Chia seed -Four tablespoons
Sugar -1 tablespoons
Cacao -Three tablespoons
Coconut milk -4 cups
Cherries, fresh-Two tablespoons
Dark chocolate, grated -¼ teaspoon
Grated coconut -¼ teaspoon
Maple syrup -One tablespoon

Instructions:
1.   Take a saucepan, add oats along with chia seeds, cocoa, and sugar, pour in the milk, and stir until mixed.
2.   Place the saucepan over medium heat, bring to boil, then lower heat to medium heat and cook for 5 to 10 minutes or until oats have softened and most of the liquid is absorbed.
3.   Spoon the oats into a bowl, top with coconut, cherries, and chocolate, drizzle with maple syrup and serve.

Creamy Whole Grain Porridge

"This porridge recipe is more of a guideline for you. Experiment with your own choice of grains, fruits, nuts, and seeds."

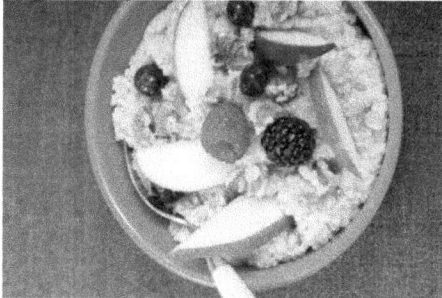

Prep Time: -5minutes -Calories: -280
Cook Time: -10minutes -Fat (g): -6.7 g
Total Time: -15minutes -Protein (g): -14 g
Servings: -1 -Carbs (g): -70 g
Ingredients:
Brown rice, cooked -1/2 cup
Sunflower seeds -1/4 cup
Pecans -1/4 cup
Raisins -Two tablespoons
Cinnamon -One teaspoon
Almond milk, unsweetened -1/4 cup
For the Topping:-
Maple syrup -1 tablespoon
Medium apple, cored, diced -1/2
Ground flax seeds -One tablespoon
Nutmeg -1/8 teaspoon
Instructions:
1.   Take a saucepan, place all the ingredients in it, except for the topping, and then stir until mixed.
2.   Place the pan over medium-low heat and cook until the rice has been cooked and mixture reaches to a porridge consistency.
3.   Spoon the porridge in a bowl, add with apple and flax seeds, sprinkle with nutmeg, and drizzle with maple syrup.
4.   Serve straight away.

Spiced Buckwheat and Chia Seed Porridge

"Buckwheat and chia seed porridge is a nutritious and enjoyable way to start your day. It will become your go-to staple for breakfast."

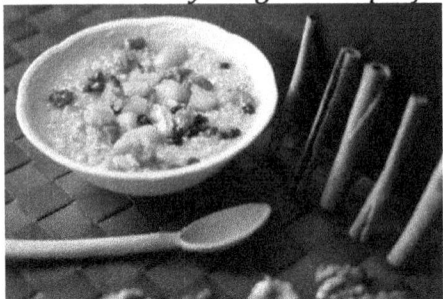

Prep Time: -6 h 10m -Calories: -241
Cook Time: -30minutes -Fat (g): -6 g
Total Time: -6 h 40m -Protein (g): -6 g
Servings: -6 -Carbs (g): -41 g
Ingredients:
Buckwheat, rinsed -1 cup
Oats, steel-cuts -½ cup
Chia seeds -Two tablespoons
Medium pear, grated with skin on-1
Medium apple, grated with skin on -1
Ground ginger-One teaspoon
Ground cinnamon -One teaspoon
Ground nutmeg-½ teaspoon
Ground cardamom -½ teaspoon
Vanilla extract, unsweetened -One teaspoon
Honey-2 tablespoons
Almond butter -Two tablespoons
Almond milk, unsweetened -2 cups
Water -2 cups
Instructions:
1.   Place oats in a bowl, add buckwheat, then pour in water and let it soak for a minimum of 6 hours or overnight.
2.   Place chia seeds in another bowl, pour in 1 cup milk and let it soak for a minimum of 6 hours or overnight.
3.   Then pour chia seeds mixture in a saucepan, pour in remaining milk, and add buckwheat and oats mixture along with remaining ingredients.
4.   Stir all the ingredients until mixed and then cook for 30 minutes over low heat until thick and creamy, stirring often.
5.   Divide porridge evenly between six bowls, top with berries and serve.

Blueberry Buckwheat Pancakes

"These gluten-free blueberry pancakes are light, fluffy, and delicious like the traditional blueberry pancakes. Make some extra pancakes, then freeze them and have them reheated whenever you want to eat them, they will still have a nice taste."

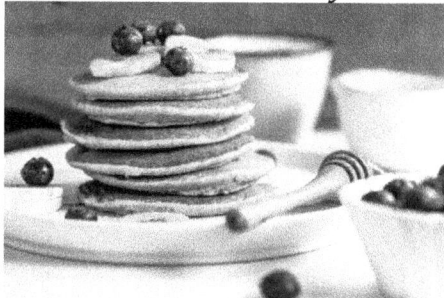

Prep Time: -10minutes -Calories: -83.5
Cook Time: -9minutes -Fat (g): -2.3 g
Total Time: -19minutes -Protein (g): -3.7 g
Servings: -8 -Carbs (g): -12 g

Ingredients:
Buckwheat flour -1 cup and two tablespoons
Baking powder -1 ½ teaspoons
Cinnamon -1/4 teaspoon
Salt -1/2 teaspoon
Brown sugar -Two tablespoons
Vanilla extract, unsweetened -1/2 teaspoon
Olive oil -One tablespoon
Plain yogurt, non-fat -1/4 cup
Egg -1
Buttermilk -1 ¼ cups
Blueberries, fresh -2 cups

Instructions:
1.   Crack the egg in a bowl, add sugar, oil, vanilla, egg, yogurt, and milk and whisk until well combined.
2.   Place the buckwheat flour in another bowl, add salt, cinnamon, and baking powder, stir until mixed, and then stir into egg mixture until incorporated and smooth batter comes together.
3.   Take a large skillet pan, place it over medium heat and when hot, pour in prepared batter, ¼ cup per pancake and then sprinkle berries on top.
4.   Cook the pancakes for 1 minute, then flip and continue cooking for 1 to 2 minutes or until the other side is nicely browned.
5.   Transfer pancakes to a plate, use the remaining batter for cooking more pancakes in the same manner, then top the pancakes with more berries, drizzle with honey and serve.

Crepes

"These gluten-free crepes take only basic pantry ingredients and are no different from regular crepes. Serve them with favorite filling."

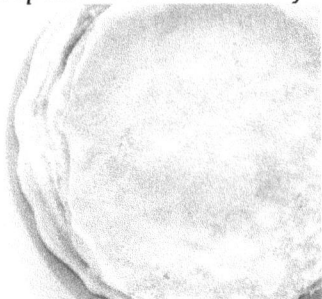

Prep Time: -10minutes -Calories: -314
Cook Time: -24minutes -Fat (g): -21 g
Total Time: -34minutes -Protein (g): -20.6 g
Servings: -6 -Carbs (g): -8.6 g

Ingredients:
Coconut flour -1 cup
Salt -¼ teaspoon
Agave nectar -Two tablespoons
Vanilla extract, unsweetened -One teaspoon
Coconut oil, melted -Two tablespoons
Olive oil -One tablespoon
Eggs -2
Almond milk, unsweetened -½ cup
Water -½ cup

Instructions:
1.   Crack the eggs in a bowl, add salt, vanilla, agave nectar, pour in milk and water, and whisk until well combined.
2.   Slowly whisk in flour until incorporated and smooth and then whisk in melted coconut oil in a steady stream until combined.
3.   Take a large frying pan, place it over medium-high heat, add olive oil and when hot, pour the batter in it, 1/3 cup per crepe, and then tilt and swirl the pan in circular to spread the batter evenly in the pan.
4.   Cook the crepe for 2 minutes until its bottom is nicely golden, then flip it and continue cooking for another 2 minutes until golden.
5.   Transfer the crepe to a plate and use the remaining batter for cooking more crepes in the same manner.
6.   Serve straight away.

Mushroom and Spinach Frittata

"This frittata features super health powers. It is abundant with fiber, anti-oxidant, and minerals that will protect your body."

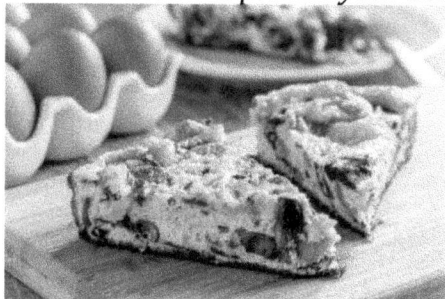

Prep Time: -10minutes -Calories: -134
Cook Time: -33minutes -Fat (g): -6 g
Total Time: -43minutes -Protein (g): -13 g
Servings: -4 -Carbs (g): -7 g
Ingredients:
Baby spinach -2 cups
Medium white onion, peeled, sliced -1
White button mushrooms, sliced -4 ounces
Almond butter, unsalted -Three tablespoons
Salt, divided -One teaspoon
Ground black pepper, divided -One teaspoon
Eggs -6
Almond milk, unsweetened -1/4 cup
Cheddar cheese, grated -1 cup
Instructions:
1.   Switch on the oven, set it to 350 degrees F, and let preheat.
2.   Crack the eggs in a bowl, whisk in milk until blended, and then whisk in cheese, ½ teaspoon each of salt and black pepper until combined.
3.   Take a skillet pan, place it over medium heat, add butter, onion, and mushrooms and cook for 5 minutes until nicely brown.
4.   Add spinach, then season with remaining salt and black pepper and cook for 1 minute, stirring constantly.
5.   Spoon the mushroom-spinach mixture into the prepared egg mixture and then stir well until combined.
6.   Take an 8-inches square baking sheet, grease it with butter, then pour in frittata mixture and bake for 25 minutes or until the frittata has puffed and the top is golden brown.
7.   When the frittata has cooked, take it out on a plate, then cut it into four squares and serve.

Spinach and Feta Frittata

"This healthy and cheesy frittata is the answer to your question 'What's for dinner?'. Anything goes with this frittata, which makes it an excellent meal for a weeknight."

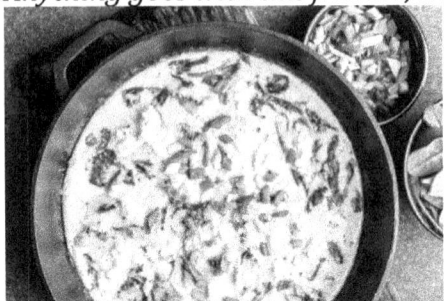

Prep Time: -10minutes -Calories: -180
Cook Time: -15minutes -Fat (g): -9.2 g
Total Time: -25minutes -Protein (g): -18.7 g
Servings: -4 -Carbs (g): -7 g

Ingredients:
Small brown onion, peeled, sliced -½
Minced garlic -One teaspoon
Baby spinach -¼ cup
Salt -¾ teaspoon
Ground black pepper -½ teaspoon
Olive oil -One teaspoon
Eggs, pastured -4
Crumbled feta cheese, low-fat -½ cup

Instructions:
1.   Set the grill and let it preheat over medium-high heat setting.
2.   Take a frying pan, place it over medium heat, add oil and when hot, add onion and cook for 3 minutes or until onions start to brown.
3.   Add spinach, cook for 2 minutes until it leaves wilts, then remove the pan from heat and let it cool.
4.   Crack the eggs in a bowl, whisk until blended, and add cooled onion-spinach mixture along with cheese, season with salt and black pepper and then whisk until well combined.
5.   Return the frying pan over medium heat, pour in egg mixture, stir gently until eggs start to set on the bottom, and then transfer the pan under the grill.
6.   Grill the frittata for 3 minutes or more until it has been thoroughly cooked, and the top is golden.
7.   When the frittata has cooked, take it out on a plate, then cut it into four squares and serve.

Scrambled Eggs

"Spinach, chia seeds and turmeric charge this egg scramble with superpowers. Not only it makes your immune system healthy, but it also supports digestion and sustains lean muscle."

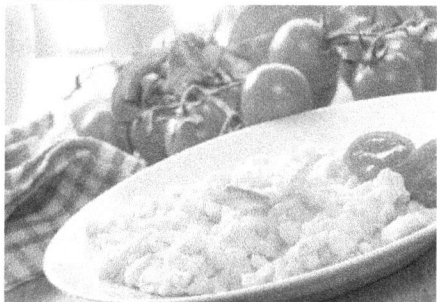

Prep Time: -5minutes -Calories: -210
Cook Time: -10minutes -Fat (g): -15 g
Total Time: -15minutes -Protein (g): -14 g
Servings: -1 -Carbs (g): -3 g

Ingredients:

Baby spinach-½ cup
Chia seeds -One teaspoon
Fresh turmeric, grated -One teaspoon
Sea salt -1/8 teaspoon
Olive oil -Two teaspoons
Coconut milk, unsweetened -Two tablespoons
Green pesto -One tablespoon
Eggs, pastured -3

Instructions:

1. Crack the eggs in a bowl, add salt, turmeric, and milk and whisk until combined.
2. Take a pan, place it over medium-low heat, add one teaspoon oil and when hot, add spinach, cook for 3 minutes until leaves have wilted, and then transfer spinach to a plate.
3. Take an 8 inches pan, grease it with remaining oil, place it over medium heat, then pour in the egg mixture and stir continuously until eggs start to set and scrambled to desire level.
4. Fold in cooked spinach and remove the pan from heat.
5. Drizzle pesto over scrambled eggs and serve straight away.

Quinoa Orange Salad

"This refreshing quinoa orange salad is super quick to make and extremely satisfying. If you already have leftover quinoa, then this salad will come together in less than 10 minutes."

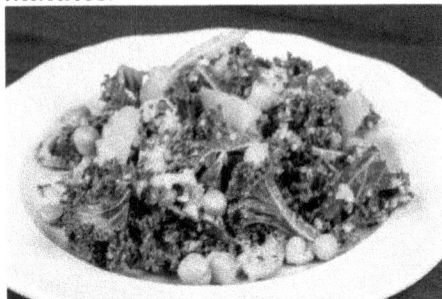

Prep Time: -40minutes -Calories: -445
Cook Time: -0minutes -Fat (g): -12.4 g
Total Time: -40minutes -Protein (g): -12.2 g
Servings: -1 -Carbs (g): -71.2 g

Ingredients:
For the Salad: -
Quinoa, cooked, cooled -1 cup
Small oranges, supremed -2
Celery rib, chopped -1
Brazil nuts, chopped -1 ½ tablespoon
Green onion, sliced -1
Fresh parsley, chopped -¼ cup
For The Dressing: -
Oranges, juiced -Of oranges used in salad
Minced garlic -1/4 teaspoon
Fresh ginger, grated -½ teaspoon
Salt -½ teaspoon
Ground black pepper -¼ teaspoon
Cinnamon -1/8 teaspoon
Lemon juice -½ teaspoon
Apple cider vinegar -One teaspoon

Instructions:
1. Prepare the salad and for this, slice each orange over a bowl into supreme, then cut supremes into bite-size pieces and place them in a bowl.
2. Add remaining ingredients for the salad and then stir until just mixed.
3. Prepare the salad dressing and for this, squeeze out the juice from the membranes of oranges, pour the juice in a food processor, add remaining ingredients for the dressing and blend until smooth.
4. Pour the dressing in the salad bowl, stir until well combined, chill the salad in the refrigerator for 30 minutes and then serve.

Lentil, Beetroot, and Hazelnut Salad

"This healthy salad features beetroot, lentil, and hazelnut that will nourish your body. Lentils are a great source of protein, beets add nice color to this salad, and ginger dressing adds incredible taste. You will love it so much!"

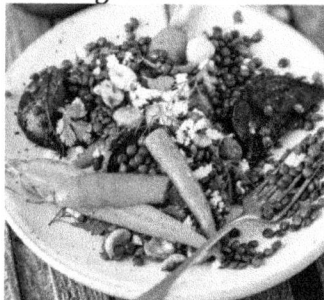

Prep Time: -10minutes -Calories: -423
Cook Time: -20minutes -Fat (g): -31 g
Total Time: -30minutes -Protein (g): -10.6 g
Servings: -3 -Carbs (g): -25.4 g

Ingredients:
For the Salad: -
Puy lentils, rinsed -1 cup
Water -2 ¾ cup
Sea salt -½ teaspoon
Beetroot, cooked, cut into small cubes -3
Spring onions, sliced -2
Hazelnuts, chopped -Two tablespoons
Fresh mint, chopped -¼ cup
Fresh parsley, roughly chopped -¼ cup
Carrot, sliced (optional) -1
For the Ginger Dressing: -
Fresh ginger, peeled, chopped -1, about ¾ inch
Olive oil -Six tablespoons
Dijon mustard -One teaspoon
Apple cider vinegar -One tablespoon

Instructions:
1.   Prepare the lentils and for this, take a saucepan, add lentils in it, pour in water, and then bring to boil.
2.   Then reduce heat to medium-low level and simmer the lentils for 15 minutes until lentils are not mushy, and cooking liquid in the pan has evaporated.
3.   Transfer cooked lentils into a bowl and then let them cool completely.
4.   Meanwhile, prepare the dressing and for this, place all its ingredients in a bowl and whisk using an immersion blender until well combined.
5.   Add remaining ingredients for the salad into lentils bowl, stir until combined, then pour in the dressing and toss until well mixed.
6.   Serve straight away.

Cauliflower Steaks with Beans

"If you are craving for beef steak, then have your craving satisfy with this impressive cauliflower steak. Beans and cherry tomatoes combined with cauliflower steaks make it a complete meal."

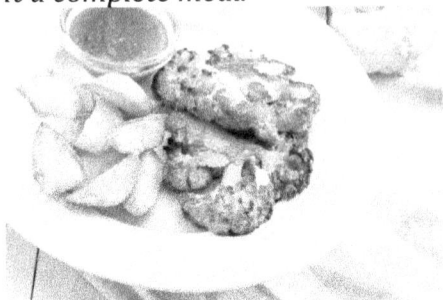

Prep Time: -15minutes -Calories: -1141
Cook Time: -40minutes -Fat (g): -77 g
Total Time: -55minutes -Protein (g): -34 g
Servings: -2 -Carbs (g): -89 g

Ingredients:
Large head of cauliflower -2 pounds
Red cherry tomatoes, halved -6 ounces
White beans, cooked -15-ounce
Green beans, trimmed -8 ounces
Panko breadcrumbs -1/3 cup
Minced garlic -1 ½ tablespoon
Salt, divided -Two teaspoons
Ground black pepper, divided -One teaspoon
Grated lemon zest -3/4 teaspoon
Chopped parsley -1/3 cup and more for serving
Olive oil, divided -1/2 cup
Grated parmesan cheese -1/4 cup
Mayonnaise -Three tablespoons
Dijon mustard -One teaspoon

Instructions:
1.   Switch on the oven, set the baking rack in the middle and upper third rack of the oven, then set it to 425 degrees F and let preheat.
2.   Meanwhile, trim the stem and remove leaves from each cauliflower, leaving the core intact, then place it on working space, core side down and cut into two 1-inch steaks by slicing from top to bottom in the center, reserving the remaining cauliflower for later use.
3.   Place cauliflower steaks on a baking sheet, brush both sides with one tablespoon oil, season with ¼ teaspoon of salt and black pepper, and then bake on the middle rack for 30 minutes until tender and nicely browned, flipping the steaks halfway through.
4.   In the meantime, place green beans in a bowl, sprinkle with ½ teaspoon salt and ¼ teaspoon black pepper, drizzle with one tablespoon oil and toss until well coated.

30

5.   Spread the green beans in another baking sheet and bake for 15 minutes in the upper third rack of oven until beans have roasted.
6.   Meanwhile, prepare the white beans and for this, place 1/3 cup parsley in a bowl, add lemon zest, remaining salt, black pepper, and oil and whisk until well combined.
7.   Transfer half of the parsley mixture in another bowl, add breadcrumbs, cheese, and mix with hands until combined.
8.   Add beans and tomatoes to the remaining parsley mixture in another bowl and then toss until well coated.
9.   Place mayonnaise in a small bowl, add mustard, and then whisk until combined, set aside until required.
10.   When cauliflower and beans have roasted, remove their baking sheet from the oven, spread mayonnaise evenly over cauliflower steaks, sprinkle evenly with ¼ cup of bread crumbs mixture and then continue roasting for 5 to 7 minutes or until the breadcrumb topping is nicely golden brown.
11.   Add white beans to the roasted green mixture, toss until well combined, and continue roasting for 5 to 7 minutes or until white beans begin to crisp.
12.   When done, divide cauliflower steaks between two plates, top with green-white beans mixture, garnish with remaining parsley and serve.

Kale Caesar Salad with Grilled Chicken Wrap

"Scrumptious kale Caesar salad as a wrap is even better as a meal on a normal night. It is so good that even if you loathe kale, please try it."

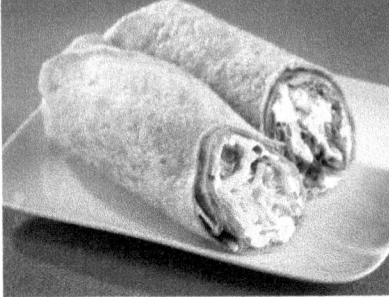

Prep Time: -10minutes -Calories: -326.3
Cook Time: -0minutes -Fat (g): -11.5 g
Total Time: -10minutes -Protein (g): -24 g
Servings: -2 -Carbs (g): -26.5 g
Ingredients:
Grilled chicken, sliced -8 ounces
Kale leaves, cut into bite-sized pieces -6 cups
Cherry tomatoes, quartered -1 cup
Minced garlic -½ tablespoon
Salt-1 ¼ teaspoon
Ground black pepper -¾ teaspoon
Dijon mustard -1/2 teaspoon
Honey-1 teaspoon
Fresh lemon juice -1/8 cup
Olive oil -1/8 cup
Shredded parmesan cheese -3/4 cup
Coddled egg -½
Large whole-grain tortillas -2
Instructions:
1.   Prepare the dressing and for this, place the coddled egg in a bowl, add mustard, garlic, and honey, drizzle with oil and lemon juice, whisk until combined and season with salt and black pepper.
2.   Then add chicken, tomatoes, and kale, sprinkle with ¼ cup cheese, pour in the dressing, and toss until coated.
3.   Place tortillas on working space, top evenly with prepared salad, sprinkle evenly with remaining cheese, and then roll up the wraps.
4.   Cut each roll in half and serve.

Grilled Sauerkraut Avocado Sandwich

"This crunchy and tangy grilled sandwich is incredibly amazing. It features healthy pumpernickel bread, creamy avocado, hummus, and tasty sauerkraut."

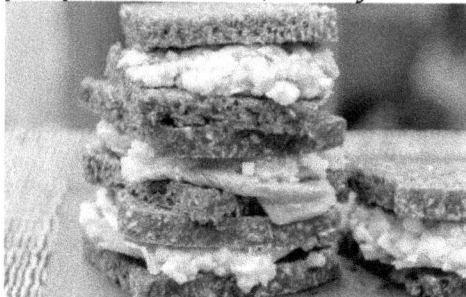

Prep Time: -10minutes -Calories: -319
Cook Time: -12minutes -Fat (g): -14 g
Total Time: -22minutes -Protein (g): -10 g
Servings: -4 -Carbs (g): -39 g

Ingredients:

Pumpernickel bread -Eight slices
Avocado, peeled, pitted-1
Almond butter, softened -Eight tablespoons
Hummus -1 cup
Sauerkraut, rinsed, and moisture squeezed out -1 cup

Instructions:

1.   Switch on the oven, set it to 450 degrees F, and let preheat.
2.   Meanwhile, spread one tablespoon butter on one side of each slice, then take a baking sheet and place four slices on it, butter-side down.
3.   Then spread half of the hummus evenly on the slices placed in the baking sheet, top with sauerkraut and avocado slices.
4.   Spread remaining hummus on the side of the remaining bread slices without butter and then place on avocado slices, hummus side down.
5.   Bake the sandwiches for 12 minutes, flipping halfway through until crispy and golden.
6.   Serve straight away.

Salmon with Smoky Chickpeas and Greens

"In this healthy meal, you will get a dose of salmon, greens, and creamy green dressing. It's a perfect dish to incorporate leafy greens into your diet."

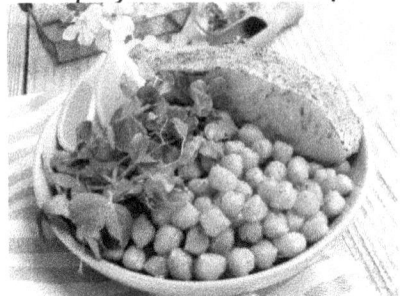

Prep Time: -10minutes -Calories: -447
Cook Time: -38minutes -Fat (g): -22 g
Total Time: -48minutes -Protein (g): -37 g
Servings: -4 -Carbs (g): -23 g

Ingredients:

Chopped kale -10 cups
Salmon, wild-caught, cut into four portions -1¼ pound
Chickpeas, cooked -15 ounces
Smoked paprika -One tablespoon
Salt, divided -½ teaspoon
Chopped chives, fresh-¼ cup and more for garnish
Ground black pepper, divided -½ teaspoon
Garlic powder -¼ teaspoon
Buttermilk -⅓ cup
Mayonnaise -¼ cup
Olive oil, divided -Two tablespoons
Water -¼ cup

Instructions:

1.   Switch on the oven, place the baking racks in the middle and upper third racks of the oven, set the oven to 425 degrees F, and let preheat.
2.   Meanwhile, prepare the dressing and for this, place ¼ teaspoon salt in a bowl, add paprika and one tablespoon oil and stir until combined.
3.   Pat dry chickpeas, add to paprika mixture, then take a rimmed baking sheet and spread the chickpeas in it in a single layer, reserving the dressing.
4.   Place the baking sheet in the upper rack of the oven and bake for 30 minutes, stirring twice.
5.   In the meantime, place mayonnaise in a blender, add chives, garlic powder, and ¼ teaspoon black pepper, pour in the milk and puree until smooth, set aside until required.
6.   Take a large skillet, add one tablespoon oil in it, place over medium heat and when hot, add kale and cook for 2 minutes.
7.   Pour in water, cook kale for another 5 minutes until tender, then remove the pan from heat and sprinkle a pinch of salt over kale.
8.   When chickpeas have roasted, push them to one side of the baking pan, then place the salmon on the other side of the baking pan and season it with remaining salt and black pepper.
9.   Return the baking sheet into the oven and bake salmon for 5 to 8 minutes or until it has thoroughly cooked.
10. When done, drizzle the remaining dressing on salmon, then sprinkle with more chives and serve with cooked kale.

Baked Tilapia

"This baked tilapia is easy and simple enough for a weeknight dinner. And the best part, it takes only 30 minutes to get on your table, from start to finish."

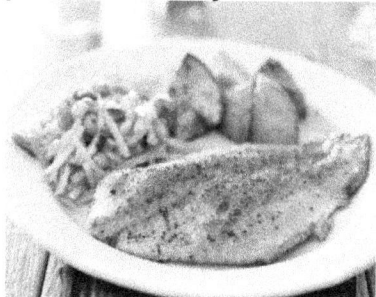

Prep Time: -10minutes -Calories: -222.4
Cook Time: -18minutes -Fat (g): -10.8 g
Total Time: -28minutes -Protein (g): -26.8 g
Servings: -4 -Carbs (g): -6.7 g

Ingredients:
Tilapia fillets -4, each about 4 ounces
Pecans chopped -1/3 cup
Panko breadcrumbs, whole grain -1/3 cup
Salt -1/8 teaspoon
Coconut sugar-1/2 teaspoon
Chopped fresh rosemary -Two teaspoons
Cayenne pepper -1/8 teaspoon
Olive oil -1 ½ teaspoon
Egg white -1

Instructions:
1.   Switch on the oven, set it to 350 degrees F, and let preheat.
2.   Meanwhile, place pecans in a bowl, add salt, sugar, rosemary, cayenne pepper and breadcrumbs, drizzle with oil and toss until well mixed.
3.   Spread the pecan mixture on a baking sheet and bake for 8 minutes or until light brown, set aside until required.
4.   In the meantime, crack the egg in a bowl and whisk until blended.
5.   Working on one fillet at a time, dip it into the egg, coat it with baked pecan mixture until evenly covered, take a large baking sheet, grease it with oil and place prepared fillets it.
6.   Sprinkle remaining pecan mixture over the fillets, pressing slightly, and then bake for 10 minutes or until tilapia is cooked.
7.   Serve straight away.

Salmon with Quinoa and Broccolini

"This quick Asian recipe brings together a vibrant and healthy salmon dinner in 30 minutes. If you don't have Broccolini, swap it with 8 ounces of broccoli florets and roast for 5 minutes."

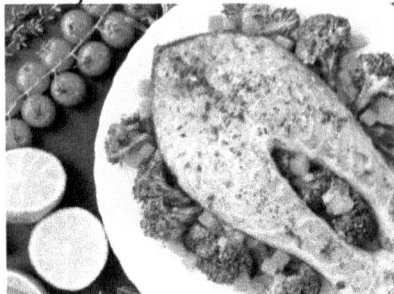

Prep Time: -5minutes -Calories: -414
Cook Time: -25minutes -Fat (g): -14 g
Total Time: -30minutes -Protein (g): -32 g
Servings: -4 -Carbs (g): -39 g

Ingredients:

Quinoa, uncooked -1 cup
Salmon fillet, wild-caught -4, each about 4-ounces
Orange juice, divided -½ cup and 1/3 cup
Scallions, sliced -2
Broccolini, trimmed -One bunch
Olive oil -One tablespoon

Ground black pepper, divided -½ teaspoon
Toasted sesame oil, divided -Three teaspoons
Garlic powder -¼ teaspoon
Black sesame seeds -One teaspoon
Grated ginger -One tablespoon
Tamari -One tablespoon
Cornstarch -One teaspoon

Instructions:

1. Cook the quinoa in ½ cup orange juice in a saucepan over medium heat until tender and thoroughly cooked.
2. Then add scallions, stir well, cover with top and set aside until required.
3. Switch on the oven, set it to 450 degrees F, and let preheat.
4. Meanwhile, place Broccolini in a bowl, season with ¼ teaspoon each of salt and black pepper, drizzle with olive oil and toss until well coated.
5. Take a rimmed baking sheet, line it with aluminum foil, spread Broccolini in it in a single layer, and bake for 8 minutes until roasted.
6. In the meantime, place remaining salt and black pepper in a small bowl, add two teaspoons sesame oil, and garlic powder, whisk until combined, and then brush this mixture generously on salmon.
7. When Broccolini has roasted, push it into one side of the pan, place the prepared salmon on the other side of the pan and continue baking for 8 minutes or until sesame is fork-tender.
8. Meanwhile, pour 1/3 cup orange juice in a heatproof bowl, add tamari, cornstarch, ginger, and 1 teaspoon sesame oil, whisk until combined, and then microwave for 1 minute at high heat setting.
9. When salmon has roasted, divide it evenly between four plates, add Broccolini and quinoa and then drizzle with prepared orange sauce.
10. Serve straight away.

Herbed Shrimps with Tomatoes

"Shrimps with tomatoes and anti-inflammatory rich herbs are perfect for boosting your digestion and health of the immune system. Adapt this recipe as per your taste and be creative."

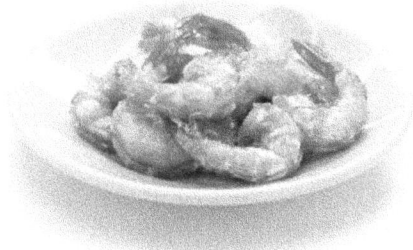

Prep Time: -10minutes -Calories: -214
Cook Time: -8minutes -Fat (g): -14.1 g
Total Time: -18minutes -Protein (g): -8 g
Servings: -2 -Carbs (g): -5.3 g

Ingredients:
Jumbo shrimp, deveined -12
Cherry tomatoes, halved -4 ounces
Coriander, chopped -Four tablespoons
Oregano, chopped -One tablespoon
Minced garlic -One teaspoon
Grated ginger -One teaspoon
Small shallot, peeled, chopped -1
Olive oil -Two tablespoons
Soy sauce -Two tablespoons
White wine -1 ounce
Almond butter, unsalted -One tablespoon
Salt-½ teaspoon
Ground black pepper -½ teaspoon

Instructions:
1. Switch on the oven, set it to 250 degrees F, and let preheat.
2. Prepare the shrimps, and for this, butterfly shrimps by slicing each shrimp in half but cutting through and then place them on a plate.
3. Season shrimps with salt and black pepper and then sprinkle with ½ tablespoon oregano and two tablespoons coriander.
4. Take a large skillet pan, add oil and when hot, add shallot, ginger, and garlic, stir until mixed and cook for 2 minutes.
5. Add shrimps in it, face down, sauté for 2 minutes per side and then remove the pan from the heat.
6. Transfer shrimps from the pan into a baking dish, sprinkle remaining oregano and coriander on shrimps, then add tomatoes, drizzle with soy sauce, stir and bake in the oven for 1 minute.
7. Then return the shrimps into the pan, add butter and cook until it sizzles.
8. Drizzle wine over shrimps and serve.

Stuffed Sweet Potato

"This recipe presents savory sweet potatoes that are stuffed with kale, avocado, and turmeric flavored chickpea scramble. This meal is beautiful, satisfying, and full of proteins, healthy fats, and antioxidants that will benefit its eater to fight with inflammation."

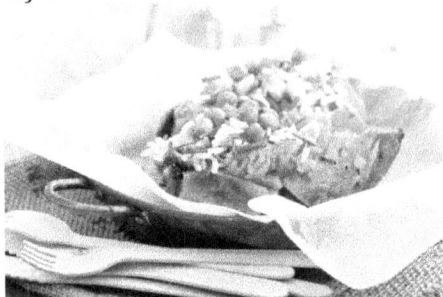

Prep Time: -10minutes -Calories: -376
Cook Time: -15minutes -Fat (g): -16 g
Total Time: -25minutes -Protein (g): -13 g
Servings: -2 -Carbs (g): -48 g

Ingredients:

For the Chickpea Scramble: -
Chickpeas, cooked -2 cups
Small red onion, peeled, diced -1/2
Minced garlic -Two tablespoons
Turmeric -One teaspoon
Sea salt -1/2 teaspoon
Olive oil -One tablespoon

Water -Two tablespoons
For the Sautéed Kale: -
Bunch of kale, de-stemmed, chopped -1
Water -Three tablespoons
For the Stuffed Sweet Potato: -
Small sweet potato, baked -1
Medium avocado -1/4

Instructions:

1.   Prepare the chickpea scramble and for this, take a pan, place it over medium heat, add oil, onion, and garlic and cook for 4 minutes or until softened.
2.   Then add chickpeas, season with salt and turmeric, drizzle with water and cook for 10 minutes or until very tender, adding more water if needed.
3.   Meanwhile, prepare the kale and for this, take another skillet pan, place it over medium heat, add kale, drizzle with water and cook for 5 minutes or more until kale has softened.
4.   When the chickpeas have cooked, remove the pan from heat, smash chickpeas with the back of a spoon, leaving 1/3 of the pea whole.
5.   Assemble the sweet potato and for this, place baked sweet potato on a plate, slice it lengthwise, top each half evenly with chickpeas scrambled, kale, and avocado and serve.

Thai Pumpkin Soup

"With just five simple ingredients, it is terribly simple to make this rich and creamy soup. Bonus – It's ready to eat in less than 15 minutes."

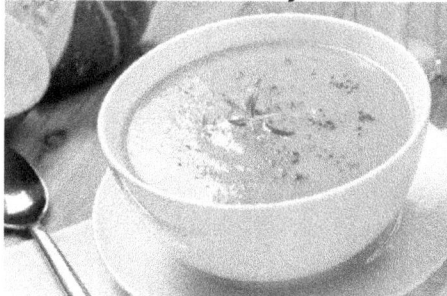

Prep Time: -5minutes -Calories: -200
Cook Time: -8minutes -Fat (g): -9 g
Total Time: -13minutes -Protein (g): -9 g
Servings: -4 -Carbs (g): -31 g

Ingredients:
Red curry paste -Two tablespoons
Vegetable broth-4 cups
Pumpkin puree -30 ounces
Coconut milk, unsweetened -1 ¾ cup
Large red chili pepper, sliced -1
Cilantro, chopped -Two tablespoons

Instructions:
1. Take a saucepan, place it over medium heat, add curry paste, cook for 1 minute until fragrant, then add pumpkin and pour in broth.
2. Stir until well mixed, cook the soup for 3 minutes or until it starts to bubbles, pour in coconut milk, reserving one tablespoon of milk, stir well and continue cooking for 3 minutes until the soup is hot.
3. Ladle the soup into bowls, drizzle with reserved coconut milk and garnish with cilantro and red chilies.
4. Serve straight away.

Cauliflower Soup

"This super simple and healthy soup features roasted cauliflower, ginger, and fennel. It is brimming with incredible flavors and probiotic-rich veggies to boost your immunity and gut health."

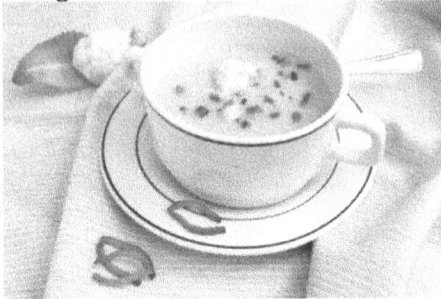

Prep Time: -10minutes -Calories: -204.5
Cook Time: -40minutes -Fat (g): -4.8 g
Total Time: -50minutes -Protein (g): -8.8 g
Servings: -4 -Carbs (g): -36.8 g

Ingredients:
Medium red onion, peeled, quartered -1
Large head of cauliflower, cut into florets -½
Fennel bulbs, cored, chopped-2
Garlic cloves, peeled -4
Turmeric powder-One teaspoon
Cinnamon -1/8 teaspoon
Black pepper -1/8 teaspoon
Tamari ,wheat-free -2 tablespoons
Sage leaves -One teaspoon
Fennel seeds -1/8 teaspoon
Hummus -Three tablespoons
Lemon -Two tablespoons
Ginger, peeled -One knob
Vegetable stock -Two ¼ cups

Instructions:
1.   Switch on the oven, set it to 400 degrees F, and let preheat.
2.   Meanwhile, take a baking tray, place cauliflower florets on it, add onion, garlic, and fennel and bake for 35 minutes or until roasted and crispy.
3.   Then transfer roasted vegetables in a food processor or blender, add remaining ingredients and pulse until smooth and creamy.
4.   Tip the blended soup into a saucepan, place it over low heat and cook for 3 to 5 minutes until thoroughly heated, taste to adjust seasoning.
5.   Ladle soup into bowls and serve.

Lentil and Chicken Soup

"Turn your leftover chicken into a hearty soup for your next dinner in no longer than 30 minutes."

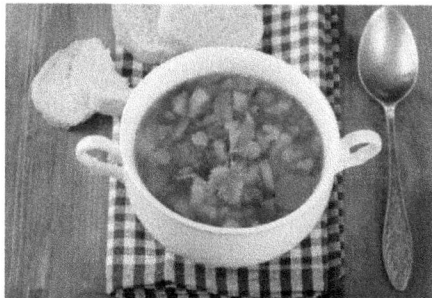

Prep Time: -10minutes -Calories: -529
Cook Time: -18minutes -Fat (g): -31 g
Total Time: -28minutes -Protein (g): -28 g
Servings: -4 -Carbs (g): -34 g
Ingredients:
Roast chicken -1
Shredded cooked chicken -1 ½ cups
French lentils 3/4 cup
Sweet potatoes, peeled, cut into 1-inch pieces -1 pound
Medium head of escarole, cut into bite-size pieces -1/2
Celery stalks, cut into ¼-inch slices -10
Minced garlic -Three tablespoons
Salt -One teaspoon
Olive oil -Two tablespoons
Chopped dill -1/2 cup
Fresh lemon juice -Two tablespoons
Water -8 cups
Instructions:
1.   Take a large pot, add roast chicken in it along with lentils and potatoes, season with one teaspoon salt, pour in water, then place the pot over high heat and bring to boil.
2.   Then reduce the heat to medium-low level and simmer the soup for 12 minutes until lentils are thoroughly cooked and potatoes are tender.
3.   Meanwhile, take a skillet pan, place it over medium-high heat, add oil and when hot, add garlic and celery and cook for 12 minutes or until tender and golden brown.
4.   When the lentils and potatoes have cooked, take out the chicken and shred its meat, about 1 ½ cup.
5.   Add shredded chicken into the pot along with celery mixture and escarole, stir until mixed, and then cook for 5 minutes until escarole has wilted.
6.   When done, remove the pot from heat, add dill and lemon juice into the soup, stir until mixed, and taste to adjust seasoning.
7.   Ladle soup into bowls and serve.

Red Pepper and Sweet Potato Soup

"This vegetarian soup is cheerfully spiced, healthy and very comforting."

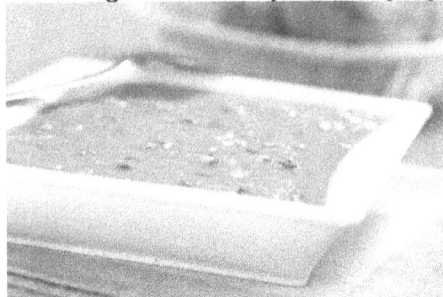

Prep Time: -10minutes -Calories: -104.4
Cook Time: -30minutes -Fat (g): -1 g
Total Time: -40minutes -Protein (g): -2.3 g
Servings: -8 -Carbs (g): -22 g

Ingredients:
Sweet potatoes, peeled, cubed -4 cups
Medium white onions, peeled, chopped -2
Roasted red peppers, chopped -12 ounces
Green chilies, diced -4 ounces
Cumin, ground -Two teaspoons
Salt -One teaspoon
Ground coriander -One teaspoon
Lemon juice -One tablespoon
Olive oil -Two tablespoons
Minced cilantro, fresh -Two tablespoons
Vegetable broth -4 cups
Cream cheese, cubed -4 ounces

Instructions:
1.   Take a large pot, place it over medium-high heat, add oil and when hot, add onion and cook for 5 minutes or until softened.
2.   Add green chilies and red pepper, season with salt, coriander, and cumin and cook for 2 minutes.
3.   Add sweet potatoes, pour in the broth, bring the soup to boil, then lower heat to medium-low level and cook for 15 minutes or until the sweet potatoes are tender, covering the pot.
4.   Then remove the pot from heat, add lemon juice and cilantro and stir until mixed.
5.   Pour half of the soup in a food processor or blender, add cream cheese and pulse until smooth and creamy.
6.   Return soup into the pot, stir well and cook for 3 minutes or until thoroughly heated, taste to adjust seasoning.
7.   Serve straight away.

Salmon with Zucchini

"Lemon and Herb crusted salmon and zucchini are the stars of this healthy meal. This food really comes together in a single pan and packed with so many flavors!"

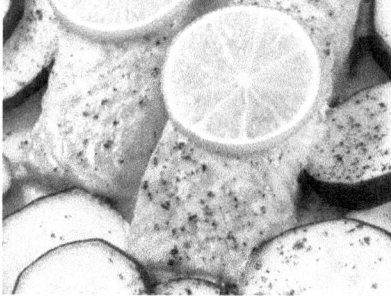

Prep Time: -10minutes -Calories: -331
Cook Time: -18minutes -Fat (g): -16.7 g
Total Time: -28minutes -Protein (g): -31 g
Servings: -4 -Carbs (g): -14.7 g

Ingredients:
Medium zucchini, chopped -4
Olive oil -Two tablespoons
Salt-1 teaspoon
Ground black pepper -½ teaspoon
Salmon fillets -4, each about 5 ounces
Chopped parsley, fresh-Two tablespoons
For The Herb Mix: -
Brown sugar -Two tablespoons
Minced garlic -One teaspoon
Dried oregano -1/2 teaspoon
Dried thyme -1/4 teaspoon
Dried rosemary -1/4 teaspoon
Salt-1 ½ teaspoons
Ground black pepper -1 ½ teaspoons
Dried dill -1/2 teaspoon
Dijon mustard -One tablespoon
Lemon juice -Two tablespoons

Instructions:
1. Switch on the oven, set it to 400 degrees F, and let preheat.
2. Meanwhile, prepare herb mix and for this, place all its ingredients in a bowl and stir until well combined.
3. Take a baking sheet, grease it with oil, and then spread with zucchini in a single layer.
4. Drizzle oil over zucchini, season with salt and black pepper, then add salmon fillets in a single layer and brush them generously with prepared herb mix.
5. Place the baking sheet into the oven and bake the zucchini and salmon for 16 to 18 minutes or until fish is fork-tender.
6. Garnish with parsley and serve.

Stuffed Red Peppers

"These Italian-styled stuffed peppers feature tasty turkey meat sauce with spinach and cheese. They are a perfect family meal. "

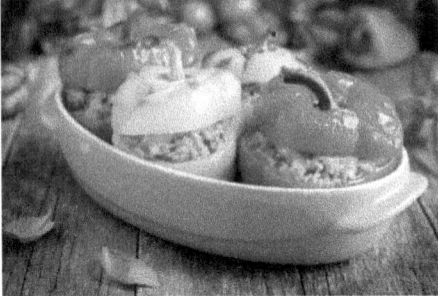

Prep Time: -10minutes -Calories: -371.1
Cook Time: -40minutes -Fat (g): -12.3 g
Total Time: -50minutes -Protein (g): -35.8 g
Servings: -3 -Carbs (g): -32.2 g

Ingredients:

Ground turkey -1 pound
Medium red bell peppers -3
Frozen chopped spinach, thawed, moisture squeezed out -½ cup
Dried basil -One teaspoon
Garlic powder -One teaspoon
Salt -½ teaspoon
Ground black pepper -½ teaspoon
Spaghetti sauce -2 cups
Grated parmesan cheese, divided -Eight tablespoons

Instructions:

1. Switch on the oven, set it to 450 degrees F, and let preheat.
2. Meanwhile, prepare the peppers, and for this, remove the stem from them by cutting around the stem, then cut each pepper in half lengthwise and discard its ribs and seeds.
3. Take a baking sheet, line it with aluminum foil, grease it with oil and place pepper halved on it, cut-side up.
4. Take a skillet pan, place it over medium-high heat, add the turkey in it and cook for 7 to 10 minutes or until thoroughly cooked.
5. Then add remaining ingredients except for cheese and spinach, stir until well mixed, cook for 2 minutes and then remove the pan from heat.
6. Add spinach into the pan along with two tablespoons cheese, stir until mixed, stuff each pepper with cooked turkey mixture, and sprinkle one tablespoon of cheese on top.
7. Bake the stuffed pepper for 30 minutes until top is nicely golden and cheese has melted.
8. Serve straight away.

Turkey and Quinoa Stuffed Bell Peppers

"These stuffed bell peppers are so good and packed with good healthy stuff. Though these bell peppers take a bit of time to prepare, the wait is so worth it."

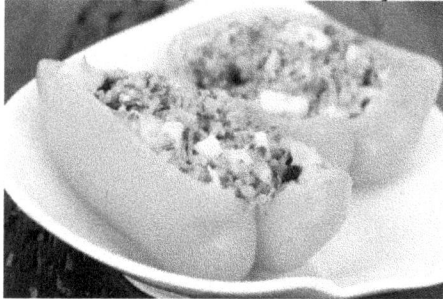

Prep Time: -15minutes -Calories: -330.3
Cook Time: -55minutes -Fat (g): -9.7 g
Total Time: -1 h 10m -Protein (g): -23 g
Servings: -6 -Carbs (g): -40 g

Ingredients:

Large yellow peppers, destemmed, cored, deseeded -3
Quinoa, cooked -1 ½ cup
Ground turkey -1.25 pound
Chopped fresh spinach -1 cup
Diced mushrooms -1 cup
Diced sweet onion -1/4 cup
Minced garlic -Two teaspoons
Olive oil -One teaspoon
Tomato sauce -1 cup
Chicken broth -1 cup
Italian cheese blend -4 ounces

Instructions:

1. Switch on the oven, set it to 400 degrees F, and let preheat.
2. Take a skillet pan, add oil and when hot, add spinach, mushroom, and onion, cook for 5 minutes, then add turkey and garlic, stir until well, and continue cooking for 10 minutes.
3. Then pour in half of the broth, add tomato sauce, stir well and simmer for 5 minutes or until most of the liquid has evaporated.
4. Meanwhile, take a baking dish, grease it with oil, cut each pepper into half, and place them in the baking dish, cut-side up.
5. Add quinoa into the cooked turkey, stir well, then spoon the mixture into pepper until stuffed and top evenly with cheese.
6. Pour the remaining broth into the base of the baking dish, cover the dish with foil and bake for 35 minutes.
7. Serve straight away.

Turkey Chili

"This slow cooker turkey chili is loaded with lean turkey, lots of vegetables, beans, and corn. It is a protein and fiber power hours and a well-rounded meal in a bowl."

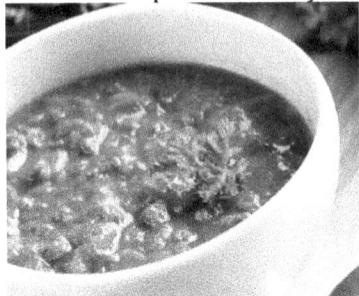

Prep Time: -5minutes -Calories: -452
Cook Time: -6 h 10m -Fat (g): -15 g
Total Time: -6 h 15m -Protein (g): -43 g
Servings: -8 -Carbs (g): -40 g

Ingredients:
Ground turkey, pastured -1 pound
Medium white onion, peeled, diced -1
Red bell pepper, cored, chopped -1
Yellow pepper, cored, chopped -1
Frozen corn -1 cup
Diced tomatoes -30 ounces
Black beans, cooked -30 ounces
Red kidney beans, cooked -30 ounces
Jalapeno peppers, sliced -16 ounces
Olive oil -One tablespoon
Red chili powder -Two tablespoons
Cumin -One tablespoon
Salt-1 ½ teaspoon
Ground black pepper -One teaspoon
Tomato sauce -30 ounces

Instructions:
1. Take a skillet pan, place it over medium heat, grease it with oil, add turkey and cook for 10 minutes or until golden brown.
2. Then transfer turkey into a slow cooker, add remaining ingredients and stir until mixed.
3. Switch on the slow cooker, shut it with its lid and let the chili cook for 6 hours at a low heat setting (for 4 hours at a high heat setting) until done.
4. Ladle chili into serving bowls, garnish with cheese and green onion and serve.

Curried Shrimp and Vegetables

"This recipe has only six ingredients and super-fast to make so it can be made on the go. If you are not in a mood of shrimps, you can make it with chicken in the same amount of time."

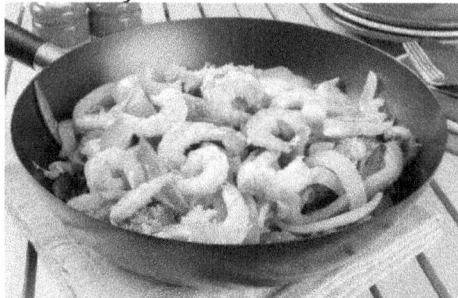

Prep Time: -5minutes -Calories: -332
Cook Time: -12minutes -Fat (g): -22.7 g
Total Time: -17minutes -Protein (g): -24 g
Servings: -4 -Carbs (g): -11.2 g

Ingredients:

Shrimp, wild-caught, peeled, deveined -1 pound
Frozen veggies-12 ounces
Medium white onion, peeled, sliced -1
Salt -One teaspoon
Ground black pepper -½ teaspoon
Curry powder -Three teaspoons
Olive oil -Three tablespoons
Coconut milk, unsweetened -1 cup

Instructions:

1. Take a skillet pan, place it over medium heat, add oil and onion and then cook for 5 minutes or until softened.
2. Meanwhile, place the vegetables in a heatproof bowl, cover it with plastic wrap and microwave for 5 minutes or more until vegetables have steamed.
3. When the onion has cooked, season with salt, black pepper, and curry seasoning, pour in milk, stir until mixed and cook for 2 minutes.
4. Then add shrimps and continue cooking for 5 minutes or until shrimps have cooked.
5. Serve shrimps with steamed vegetables.

Salmon & Brussels Sprouts

"Salmon with garlic and Brussel Sprouts, flavored with oregano is a simple enough meal for a busy weeknight. And, not to mention, it has lots of omega-3 fatty acids that will reduce the inflammation."

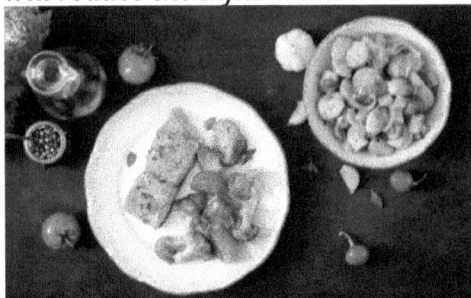

Prep Time: -10minutes -Calories: -334
Cook Time: -25minutes -Fat (g): -15 g
Total Time: -35minutes -Protein (g): -33 g
Servings: -6 -Carbs (g): -10 g

Ingredients:
Salmon fillet, wild-caught, skinned -2 pounds
Large garlic cloves, peeled, divided -14
Chopped oregano, fresh, divided -Two tablespoons
Salt, divided -One teaspoon
Ground black pepper, divided -¾ teaspoon
Brussels sprouts, trimmed, sliced -6 cups
White wine -¾ cup
Olive oil -¼ cup
Lemon wedges -As needed

Instructions:
1.   Switch on the oven, set it to 450 degrees F, and let preheat.
2.   Meanwhile, mince two cloves of garlic, add it in a small bowl along with ¼ teaspoon salt, one tablespoon oregano, and ¼ teaspoon black pepper, pour in the oil and stir until combined.
3.   Cut the remaining garlic in half, add them in a large bowl along with Brussels sprouts, drizzle with three tablespoons of the prepared oil mixture and toss until well coated.
4.   Spread Brussel sprouts in a large roasting pan and then roast for 15 minutes, stirring halfway through.
5.   Meanwhile, pour wine into the remaining oil mixture and then whisk until combined.
6.   When the sprouts have baked, stir them, then cut salmon into six pieces and place them on top of Brussel sprouts.
7.   Drizzle with oil-wine mixture over salmon, sprinkle with remaining salt and oregano, and black pepper and continue baking for 5 to 10 minutes or until salmon is thoroughly cooked.
8.   Serve salmon and sprouts with lemon wedges.

Mediterranean Tuna Salad

"If you are out of whole-grain bread, then this tomato stuffed tuna salad is here to calm down your hunger. It is light, fresh, creamy, and so tasty that the flavor will kick your taste buds."

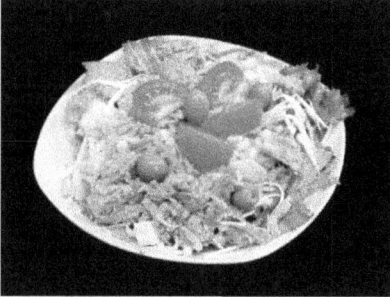

Prep Time: -10minutes -Calories: -150
Cook Time: -0minutes -Fat (g): -9 g
Total Time: -10minutes -Protein (g): -13 g
Servings: -2 -Carbs (g): -3 g

Ingredients:
Cooked tuna -10 ounces
Chopped Kalamata olives -1/4 cup
Large tomatoes -2
Chopped red peppers, fire-roasted -Two tablespoons
Minced red onion -Two tablespoons
Capers -One tablespoon
Chopped basil, fresh -Two tablespoons
Lemon juice -One tablespoon
Salt-½ teaspoon
Ground black pepper -1/3 teaspoon
Mayonnaise -1/4 cup

Instructions:
1. Prepare the salad and for this, place all the ingredients in a large bowl, except for tomatoes and then stir until combined.
2. Cut each tomato, don't cut all the way through, then open the tomatoes and scoop prepared salad into its center.
3. Serve straight away.

Salmon & Cauliflower Rice Bowl

"This meal bowl is loaded with anti-inflammatory and pro-biotics rich foods that are keys to heal your gut and calm inflammation. And not to mention, it tastes incredible!"

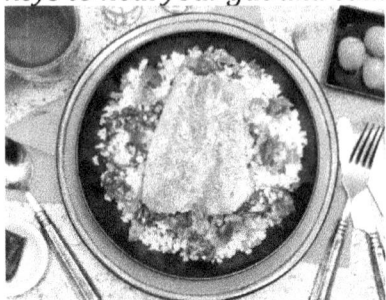

Prep Time: -10minutes -Calories: -470
Cook Time: -35minutes -Fat (g): -32 g
Total Time: -45minutes -Protein (g): -15 g
Servings: -2 -Carbs (g): -34 g

Ingredients:

Salmon fillets, wild-caught -2
Brussels sprouts, halved -12
Kale, rinsed, shredded -One bunch
Medium head of cauliflower, riced -½
Olive oil -Three tablespoons
Curry powder -One teaspoon
Himalayan salt -½ teaspoon
For the Marinade: -
Tamari sauce -¼ cup
Dijon mustard -One teaspoon
Sesame oil -One teaspoon
Maple syrup -One teaspoon
Sesame seeds -One tablespoon

Instructions:

1.   Switch on the oven, set it to 350 degrees F, and let preheat.
2.   Meanwhile, take a baking sheet, add halved Brussel sprouts, drizzle with one tablespoon oil, season with salt, toss until well coated and bake in the oven for 20 minutes until roasted.
3.   In the meantime, prepare the marinade and for this, place all its ingredients in a bowl, whisk until combined, and set aside until required.
4.   When Brussel sprouts have roasted, transfer them to a plate, place salmon fillets in the baking sheet, drizzle with prepared marinade and continue roasting for 15 minutes or until salmon is fork-tender.
5.   Meanwhile, take a skillet pan, place it over medium-high heat, add one tablespoon oil and kale and cook for 3 minutes until sauté, set aside until required.
6.   Return the pan over heat, add remaining oil and cauliflower rice, season with salt and curry powder, stir until mixed and cook for 3 minutes or until sauté.
7.   When salmon has cooked, divide it and Brussel sprouts evenly between two bowls, add cauliflower rice and kale and serve.

Lettuce Wraps with Smoked Trout

"The combination of smoked trout, cucumber, carrots dressed in a sweet and hot sauce is a handheld treat. These wraps need simple ingredients and are easy to make."

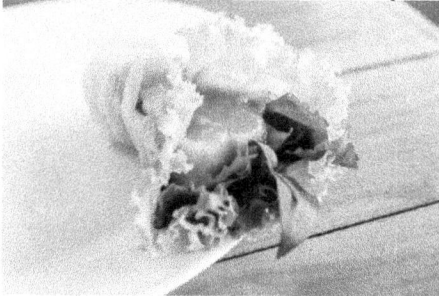

Prep Time: -40minutes -Calories: -423
Cook Time: -0minutes -Fat (g): -12 g
Total Time: -40minutes -Protein (g): -33 g
Servings: -4 -Carbs (g): -60 g

Ingredients:
Medium carrots, peeled -2
Diced grape tomatoes -1 cup
Cucumber, unpeeled-1/2
Shallots, peeled, thinly sliced -1/4 cup
Jalapeño chilies, thinly sliced with seeds-1/4 cup
Medium leaves of romaine lettuce-16
Smoked trout fillets, cut into bite-size pieces -2 cups
Mint leaves, fresh -1/2 cup
Basil leaves, fresh -1/2 cup
Lime juice-Two tablespoons
Coconut sugar -One tablespoon
Fish sauce-One tablespoon
Asian sweet chili sauce -1/3 cup
Peanuts, dry-roasted, chopped, lightly salted -1/4 cup

Instructions:
1.   Shave cucumber and carrots into ribbons by using a vegetable peeler, cut the ribbons into 3-inches pieces, then cut into strips about matchstick-size and place in a bowl.
2.   Add jalapeno pepper and shallots, sprinkle with sugar, drizzle with fish sauce and lime juice, toss until well coated and let it marinate at room temperature for 30 minutes.
3.   Then add tomatoes and trout into the vegetables, toss until well mixed, then transfer the mixture into a strainer, drain it well and return it into the bowl.
4.   Add basil and mint into the vegetable-trout mixture and toss until mixed.
5.   Assemble the wraps and for this, place lettuce leaves on a large plate, evenly scoop with prepared vegetable-trout salad, drizzle with chili sauce and then sprinkle with peanuts.
6.   Serve straight away.

Avocado Pesto Zoodles with Salmon

"Zucchini noodles with salmon and avocado pesto is a nutritious alternative to pasta. It is really light, yet super filling meal, with lots of omega-3s."

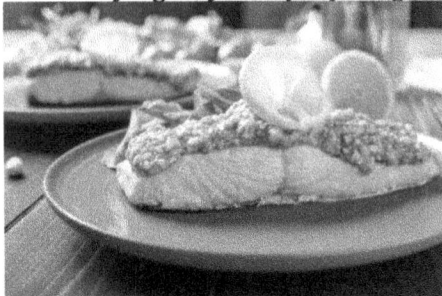

Prep Time: -10minutes -Calories: -410
Cook Time: -20minutes -Fat (g): -22 g
Total Time: -30minutes -Protein (g): -33 g
Servings: -4 -Carbs (g): -23 g

Ingredients:
Frozen salmon steaks, defrosted -2
Large zucchini -1
Avocado, pitted -1
Grated parmesan cheese -1/4 cup
Basil pesto-1 tablespoon
Lemon juice -Five tablespoons
Ground black pepper-1 ½ teaspoon

Instructions:
1.   Switch on the oven, set it to 350 degrees F, and let preheat.
2.   Take a baking sheet, place salmon steaks on it, drizzle with two tablespoon lemon juice, season with 1 teaspoon black pepper, then bake for 20 minutes until salmon is fork-tender.
3.   Meanwhile, make noodles of the zucchini by using a spiralizer and set aside until required.
4.   Place avocado in a bowl, mash it well with a fork, add two tablespoon lemon juice, pesto, and remaining black pepper, stir well, and set aside until required.
5.   Divide zucchini noodles evenly between serving plates, top with prepared avocado mixture and baked salmon, and then sprinkle with parmesan cheese.
6.   Serve straight away.

Korean Mackerel

"Mackerel is a perfect oily fish to treat your inflammation. Moreover, it pairs well with bold and strong-flavored ingredients."

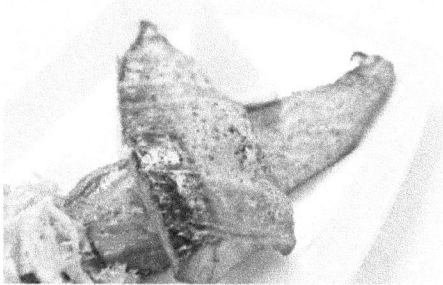

Prep Time: -10minutes -Calories: -221
Cook Time: -30minutes -Fat (g): -7 g
Total Time: -40minutes -Protein (g): -34 g
Servings: -4 -Carbs (g): -4 g

Ingredients:

Whole mackerel, wild-caught, cleaned, tails left on, butterflied -2, each 1 ½ pounds
Korean Chile paste -Two tablespoons
Grated ginger, fresh -One teaspoon
Soy sauce -One tablespoon
Apple cider vinegar -Two teaspoons
Olive oil -One tablespoon

Instructions:

1. Prepare the paste and for this, place ginger in a small bowl, add Chile paste, vinegar, and soy sauce and whisk until combined.
2. Butterfly each fish, open it, and then place the fishes in a baking sheet.
3. Then spread the marinade over the fish, reserving two tablespoons for later use and marinade for a minimum of 30 minutes.
4. When ready to cook, set the grill and let preheat over medium heat.
5. Brush the grilling rack with oil generously, place marinated fish on it, flesh side down, and grill for 3 minutes.
6. Then flip the fish, spread with reserve paste, and continue grilling for 4 minutes until opaque.
7. Serve straight away.

Salmon Cakes

"These salmon cakes are bursting with the flavors and nutrition of Mediterranean ingredients, making it a perfect anti-inflammatory food."

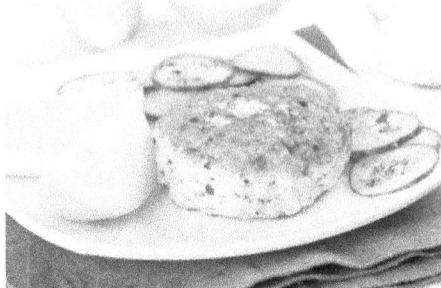

Prep Time: -15minutes -Calories: -243
Cook Time: -16minutes -Fat (g): -8.5 g
Total Time: -31minutes -Protein (g): -18 g
Servings: -6 -Carbs (g): -28.2 g

Ingredients:

For the Salmon Cakes: -One tablespoon
Cooked red salmon, wild-caught, skinless, bones removed -14.75 ounces
Cooked chickpeas -15 ounces
Panko breadcrumbs, whole-grain -1 cup
Olives, sliced -¼ cup
Chopped parsley, fresh -½ cup
Lime juice -Two tablespoons
Hot sauce -One teaspoon

Cumin, ground -½ teaspoon
Salt -¼ teaspoon
Egg whites, beaten -2
Olive oil -One tablespoon
For the Sauce: -
Diced cucumber -2/3 cup
Yogurt -2/3 cup
Dried dill -¼ teaspoon
Minced garlic -One tablespoon

Instructions:

1. Prepare the sauce and for this, place all its ingredients in a bowl, stir until well mixed and set aside until required.
2. Prepare the salmon cakes and for this, place chickpeas in a bowl, mash them partially with a fork, add olives, salmon, and breadcrumbs and stir until mixed.
3. Crack eggs in a bowl, add salt, cumin, and parsley, pour in lime juice and hot sauce and whisk until blended.
4. Add the egg mixture into salmon, stir until well combined, and then shape the mixture into twelve patties, each about 3/4-inch thick.
5. Take a large skillet pan, place it over medium-high heat, add 1 ½ teaspoon oil and when hot, add salmon cakes in a single layer and cook for 4 minutes per side until golden.
6. Transfer the cooked salmon cakes to a plate, add remaining oil into the pan, then add remaining salmon cakes and cook them in the same manner.
7. Serve salmon cakes with prepared sauce.

Chocolate Chia Hemp Pudding

"This chocolate, chia, and hemp seeds pudding is packed with protein, minerals, vitamins, antioxidants and plenty of omega-3 fatty acids to fight off inflammation. Moreover, this pudding recipe is customizable, so be creative with it.

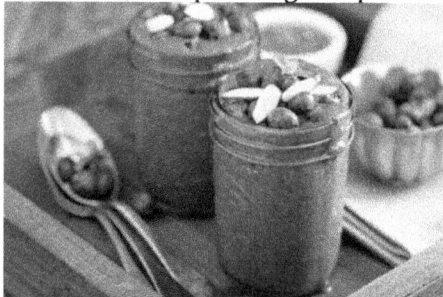

Prep Time: -4 h 5m -Calories: -113.7
Cook Time: -0minutes -Fat (g): -10 g
Total Time: -4 h 5m -Protein (g): -5.4 g
Servings: -1 -Carbs (g): -12.5 g
Ingredients:
Chia seeds -Two tablespoons
Hemp seeds -Two tablespoons
Cacao powder -One tablespoon
Small dates, pitted-6
Almond milk, unsweetened -1/2 cup
For the Topping:-
Strawberry, sliced -2
Walnuts, chopped -One teaspoon
Pumpkin seeds -½ teaspoon
Instructions:
1.   Place all the ingredients in a food processor or blender and pulse until well combined.
2.   Tip the pudding in a bowl and then refrigerate for a minimum for 4 hours or until pudding is set and chilled.
3.   When ready to serve, stir the pudding, top the pudding with sliced berries, walnuts, and pumpkin seeds and serve.

Blueberry Almond Chia Pudding

"This chia pudding is a perfect recipe for make-ahead breakfast or dessert. This pudding couldn't be easier, and you will just need six ingredients."

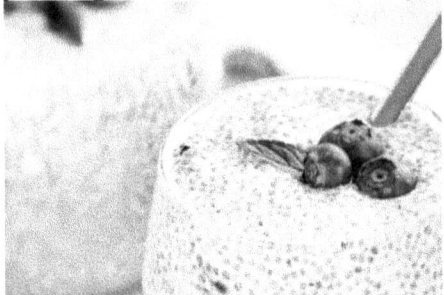

Prep Time: -8 h 10m -Calories: -229
Cook Time: -0minutes -Fat (g): -11 g
Total Time: -8 h 10m -Protein (g): -6 g
Servings: -1 -Carbs (g): -30 g

Ingredients:
Fresh blueberries, divided -½ cup
Chia seeds -Two tablespoons
Maple syrup -Two teaspoons
Almond extract, unsweetened -⅛ teaspoon
Slivered almonds, toasted, divided -One tablespoon
Almond milk, unsweetened-½ cup

Instructions:
1.   Add chia seeds in a bowl, add maple syrup, pour in the milk, and stir until well mixed.
2.   Cover the bowl and then refrigerate it for a minimum for 8 hours or until pudding is set and chilled.
3.   When ready to serve, stir the pudding, then spoon half of the pudding in a serving bowl, and top with half of almonds and blueberries.
4.   Add remaining pudding over berries, then top with remaining almonds and blueberries and serve.

Hemp Protein Bars

"This no-bake healthy bars only need six ingredients to come together. Hemp seeds are high in omega-3, iron, and manganese, which is good for tendon pain and red blood cell respectively. And therefore, all of these factors of hemp seeds make the protein bars excellent anti-inflammatory food."

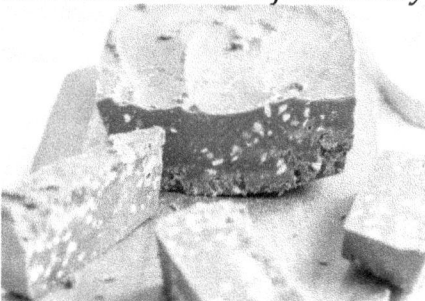

Prep Time: -1 h and 5m -Calories: -231
Cook Time: -0minutes -Fat (g): -10 g
Total Time: -1 h and 5m -Protein (g): -8 g
Servings: -14 -Carbs (g): -28 g

Ingredients:

 Almonds -1 cup
Soft pitted dates -2 cups
Hemp protein powder -1/2 cup
Cinnamon -One tablespoon
Almond butter-1/2 cup
Maple syrup -Two tablespoons

Instructions:

1.   Place almonds in a food processor and then process until nuts have broken down.
2.   Then add dates, continue processing until blended, add remaining ingredients, and continue blending until the thick dough comes together.
3.   Take a small square baking pan, line it with parchment paper, add the nut mixture, then spread it evenly and press into the pan.
4.   Place the pan in the freezer and let chill for 60 minutes or more until hard.
5.   Then cut the mixture into fourteen bars and serve.

Cranberry-Almond Granola Bars

"This granola bar recipe is nutritious and versatile. Feel free to use your choice of ingredients as per your taste and make them easily at home."

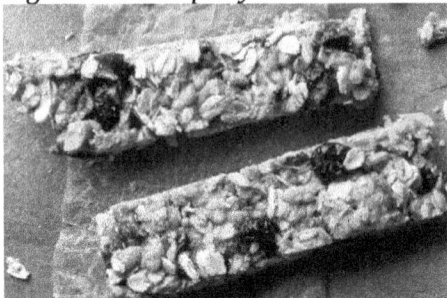

Prep Time: -50minutes -Calories: -161
Cook Time: -35minutes -Fat (g): -7 g
Total Time: -1 h 25m -Protein (g): -3 g
Servings: -24 -Carbs (g): -23 g
Ingredients:
Rolled oats, old-fashioned -3 cups
Brown rice cereal -1 cup
Dried cranberries -1 cup
Almonds, toasted, chopped -½ cup
Pecans, toasted, chopped -½ cup
Salt -¼ teaspoon
Brown rice syrup-⅔ cup
Almond butter -½ cup
Vanilla extract, unsweetened -One teaspoon
Instructions:
1.   Switch on the oven, set it to 325 degrees F, and let preheat.
2.   Meanwhile, place oats in a bowl, add berries, pecans, cereal, and almonds, sprinkle with salt, and stir until mixed.
3.   Place butter in a small heatproof bowl, add rice syrup and vanilla and microwave for 30 seconds at a high heat setting.
4.   Add the butter mixture into pats mixture and then stir evenly until well combined.
5.   Take a 9 by 13 inches baking pan, line it with parchment paper, grease it with oil, then spoon in oats mixture, spread it evenly by pressing into the pan and bake for 35 to 35 minutes until edges start to golden brown and middle is firm.
6.   Let the granola cool in the pan for 10 minutes, then pull the parchment paper to transfer the granola to a cutting board and cut into twenty-four pieces.
7.   Transfer the granola bars onto a wire rack and then let cool for 30 minutes.
8.   Serve straight away.

Chocolate Chip Granola Bars

"These no-bake chocolate chip granola bars need just a few simple pantry ingredients. You can have them as a snack or dessert because they are so good."

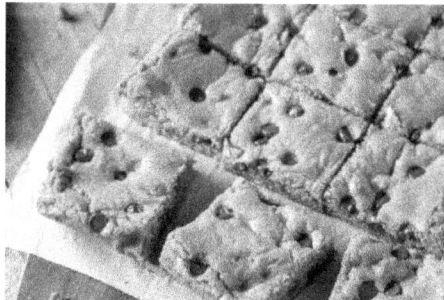

Prep Time: -3 h 25m -Calories: -100
Cook Time: -0minutes -Fat (g): -3.5 g
Total Time: -3 h 25m -Protein (g): -1 g
Servings: -10 -Carbs (g): -17 g

Ingredients:

Raisins-2 cups
Pure maple syrup -Three tablespoons
Almond butter-1/2 cup
Oats-2 cups
Sunflower seeds -1 cup
Chocolate chips, dairy-free -1/2 cup

Instructions:

1.   Place raisins in a bowl, pour in hot water to cover them, let them soak for 15 minutes and then drain them.
2.   Place raisins in a blender or food processor, pulse until raisins break down, then add remaining ingredients except for chocolate chips and blend until dough starts to come together.
3.   Then add chocolate chips, pulse until just mixed, and then scoop the mixture into a baking pan lined with parchment sheet.
4.   Spread the granola mixture evenly and then refrigerate for 3 hours or until set.
5.   Then pull out the parchment sheet to transfer the granola to a cutting board and cut it into ten bars.
6.   Serve straight away.

Purple Fruit Salad

"Grapes, berries, juicy plumps, and a zesty salad dressing brings together this rainbow and crowd-pleasing salad."

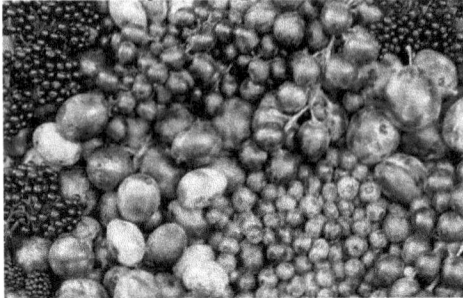

Prep Time: -4 h 10m -Calories: -77
Cook Time: -0minutes -Fat (g): -1 g
Total Time: -4 h 10m -Protein (g): -3 g
Servings: -8 -Carbs (g): -14 g

Ingredients:
For the Salad: -
Black grapes, halved, seedless -2 cups
Blueberries, halved-2 cups
Plums, diced -2 cups
For Fruit Salad Dressing: -
Yogurt, low-fat -1 cup
Lime zest -¾ tablespoon
Lime juice -¾ tablespoon
Coconut sugar -2 ½ teaspoons

Instructions:
1.   Prepare the dressing and for this, place all its ingredients in a bowl, whisk until well combined, and set aside.
2.   Prepare the salad and for this, place all its ingredients in a bowl and stir until just mixed.
3.   Add the dressing, toss until well coated, and refrigerate for a minimum of 4 hours until chilled.
4.   Serve straight away.

Winter Fruit Salad

"Pears, persimmons, and grapes feature in this vibrant and heavenly salad. This healthy fruit salad is perfect for a dessert, particularly on holiday."

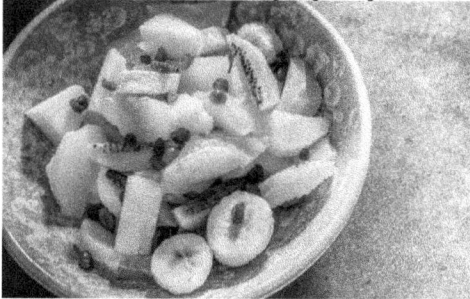

Prep Time: -10minutes -Calories: -91.6
Cook Time: -0minutes -Fat (g): -5.1 g
Total Time: -10minutes -Protein (g): -1.8 g
Servings: -4 -Carbs (g): -12 g
Ingredients:
For the Salad: -
Fuyu persimmons, 1-inch cubed -1 cup
Banana, sliced -1 cups
Kiwifruit, sliced -1/2 cup
Pecans, slivered -1/4 cup
For the Dressing: -
Olive oil -1 tablespoon
Peanut oil -One tablespoon
Pomegranate-flavored vinegar -1 tablespoon
Agave nectar -Two tablespoons
Salt -1/16 teaspoon
Instructions:
1.   Prepare the dressing and for this, place all its ingredients in a bowl and whisk until combined.
2.   Prepare the salad and for this, place all its ingredients in a bowl, except for pecans and stir until just mixed.
3.   Add the dressing, toss until well coated, and then toss in pecans until mixed.
4.   Serve straight away.

www.ingramcontent.com/pod-product-compliance
Lightning Source LLC
Chambersburg PA
CBHW080630030426
42336CB00018B/3142

* 9 7 8 1 6 4 9 8 4 7 7 2 0 *